MW01121253

The forensic mental health system in Ontario

An information guide

Shannon Bettridge, MA

Howard Barbaree, PhD, C.Psych.

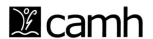

Centre for Addiction and Mental Health
Centre de toxicomanie et de santé mentale
Un Centre collaborateur de l'Organisation panaméricaine de la Santé
et de l'Organisation mondiale de la Santé

National Library of Canada Cataloguing in Publication

Bettridge, Shannon

The forensic mental health system in Ontario : an information guide /
Shannon Bettridge, Howard Barbaree.

1. Forensic psychiatry–Ontario. I. Barbaree, Howard, 1946-
II. Centre for Addiction and Mental Health III. Title.

RA1151.B48 2004 614'.15'09713 C2004-901321-1

ISBN: 978-1-77052-627-3 (PRINT)
ISBN: 978-1-77052-628-0 (PDF)
ISBN: 978-1-77052-629-7 (HTML)
ISBN: 978-1-77052-630-3 (ePUB)

PM031

Printed in Canada

Copyright © 2004, 2008, Centre for Addiction and Mental Health

No part of this work may be reproduced or transmitted in any form or by any means
electronic or mechanical, including photocopying and recording, or by any information
storage and retrieval system without written permission from the publisher—except for
a brief quotation (not to exceed 200 words) in a review or professional work.

This publication may be available in other formats. For information about
alternate formats, or other CAMH publications, or to place an order, please contact
Sales and Distribution:
Toll-free: 1 800 661-1111
Toronto: 416 595-6059
E-mail: publications@camh.net
Online store: http://store.camh.net

Web site: www.camh.net

Disponible en français sous le titre :
Le système ontarien de services psychiatriques médico-légaux : Guide d'information

This guide was produced by the following:
Development: Andrew Johnson, CAMH
Editorial: Sue McCluskey, CAMH; Sally McBeth, Clear Language and Design;
  Nick Gamble, CAMH
Design: Nancy Leung, CAMH
Print production: Christine Harris, CAMH

3973l / 01-2012 / PM031j23

Contents

Acknowledgments

The Centre for Addiction and Mental Health (CAMH) wishes to acknowledge the patients, families and professionals who helped to create this resource. Their expertise in the forensic mental health system has helped to make this an informative resource. Their commitment to providing clear, accessible information to those who need it deserves our thanks. Any shortcomings in this resource are solely the responsibility of CAMH.

We acknowledge the contribution of Dr. Sandy Simpson, Clinical Director, and other staff of CAMH's Law and Mental Health Program, who reviewed this text in 2011 and made numerous small but significant improvements.

1 Introduction

This guide will help you learn about the forensic mental health system in Ontario. If you, or someone you know, has a mental illness and has come into contact with the law, you should read this guide.

What is the forensic mental health system?

The **mental health system** is the network of people and services that care for people with mental illness. The **criminal justice system** includes the courts, the institutions and the professionals that deal with people accused or convicted of crimes. If you have a mental illness and you come into contact with the law, you could become involved with the forensic mental health system.

In this guide, "**forensic**" means "connected to the law or the courts." "Mental illness" is a very broad term that can mean many things. People who have symptoms of a mental illness sometimes have trouble knowing what is real. Sometimes they hear or see things that other people don't hear or see. Sometimes they have thoughts or beliefs that are not logical or true, but they can't stop thinking about them. Mental illness includes psychotic illnesses such as schizophrenia and mood problems such as bipolar disorder and major depression. Some people have what is called a "**dual diagnosis.**" This refers to a person who has both a mental illness and an intellectual disability (also known as a "developmental delay" or "mental retardation"). Both people with a mental illness alone and people with a dual diagnosis can enter the forensic mental health system.

People who have a mental illness and who come into contact with the law have special needs. The mental health system or the criminal justice system alone cannot always meet those needs. The forensic mental health system is the place where the mental health system and the criminal justice system meet.

The forensic mental health system can be confusing and frightening for people who have a mental illness. The legal system can be intimidating. Your freedom may be limited. It may be hard to understand why so many people suddenly become so involved in your life. These people may include police, lawyers, judges, doctors and members of review boards. This book is designed to help you understand what is happening.

How to use this guide

The forensic mental health system is very complex. You may have to read parts of this guide a few times. As you move through the different stages of the system, certain parts of this guide will make more sense or become more important for you.

The guide explains:

• what the forensic mental health system is

- who is involved
- what happens once you are in the system
- what happens when you leave the system.

> In this guide, the word "family" refers to relatives, partners, friends or anyone who cares about a person, no matter what the actual relationship is.
>
> Words printed in **bold type** are explained in a glossary at the back of the guide.

Where to go for more information

You may have questions about the forensic mental health system that this guide does not answer. If so, check the list of resources at the back of this booklet.

This guide is not a legal text and does not replace the expertise of a lawyer. The goal of this guide is simply to describe the way the forensic mental health system typically works in Ontario. If you have more questions about the legal system, talk to a lawyer.

You can also talk to a psychiatrist, social worker or nurse if you do not understand what is happening to you in the forensic mental health system.

Why do we have a forensic mental health system?

Society believes it is unfair to punish people for a criminal act if people have a mental illness that:

• prevents them from understanding what they have done, or
• prevents them from realizing what the result of their actions will be.

The restrictions and rules of the forensic mental health system may be hard to get used to, but the main goal is rehabilitation. This means improving your mental health and helping you to live successfully in the community.

> The role of the forensic mental health system is not to punish. It is to help rehabilitate and reintegrate people into the community.

Myths about mental illness

There is a myth that all people with mental illness are dangerous or violent. This is not true. Mental illness is like physical illness—it can affect anybody. Some people with mental illness can be violent. So can people who do not have a mental illness.

Only some people in the forensic mental health system are there because they have been violent. Many non-violent offences also bring people into the forensic mental health system. These offences may include mischief, theft or drug use. Those who have committed a violent offence often did so when they were ill. They may not have understood what they were doing or what would happen as a result.

People who have a mental illness have to live with many negative attitudes that others have about them. These ideas are sometimes called "stigma." Stigma leads to discrimination, disrespect and much worse. People in the forensic mental health system feel they have a "double stigma" when others unfairly label them as "dangerous."

The people who work in the forensic mental health system know about the problem of stigma. They are committed to treating everyone with respect and dignity.

2 Who works in the forensic mental health system?

The forensic mental health system involves people who know about both the mental health and the criminal justice systems.

Police

Police make the community safe and enforce the law. Neighbours or strangers might call the police if they feel frightened by someone, or when they think a crime has been committed. Sometimes family members call the police as a way of getting help for their loved one, who they feel needs more care than he or she is currently getting.

Getting people "help"—treatment—is not always something the police can do. Please read the section "How do people enter the forensic mental health system?" on page 13 for more information.

Defence counsel

If you have been arrested, you should contact a lawyer as soon as you can. This person becomes your defence counsel. Your defence counsel can tell you what might happen to you once you have been arrested. You can ask for advice about what you should do.

If you don't have a lawyer and need to find one, or if you don't have a lawyer and need to apply for Legal Aid, read the section "What happens after a person is arrested?" on page 14 for more information.

Duty counsel

Duty counsel are lawyers who work in the court. They will help you if you do not yet have your own lawyer. They are paid by Legal Aid and their help is free. Duty counsel can help with basic legal advice and court proceedings. However, they work with many people. They will not be able to get to know you or your case well. Often there is a different duty counsel in the courthouse every day. You will likely still need a lawyer to represent you.

Crown counsel

This person is the lawyer for the Crown, representing society and the public. Crown counsel is sometimes called "the prosecutor," "Crown attorney" or simply "the Crown." The legal system is "adversarial." This means that two different sides of the case will be presented—your side, argued by your lawyer, and the Crown's side, argued by Crown counsel. Crown counsel must show evidence of the alleged crime and present all the facts fairly.

Judge

The judge (and sometimes a jury of 12 citizens) listens to evidence given by your defence counsel and the Crown counsel.

The judge decides the following:

- If you are in jail, the judge decides if you should be granted bail. With bail, you can live in the community until your court date. A justice of the peace may decide this instead of a judge.
- The judge can decide if your mental health should be assessed.
- Based on the assessment of your mental health, the judge decides if you are Fit to Stand Trial.
- The judge (and sometimes a jury) decides if you are Not Criminally Responsible (NCR) because of your mental illness.
- If you are criminally responsible, the judge (and sometimes a jury) can find you guilty.
- If you are found guilty, the judge decides what your sentence will be.

Court support workers and diversion programs

Some courts have a **Court Support Program.** You might not know what kind of help you need or what services are in your area. Court Support Workers can help link you up with those services.

Court Support Workers are also involved in **diversion** programs. These programs are for people who have been charged with a minor offence. The idea is to keep people who have a serious mental illness and have also committed a minor offence out of the criminal justice system. Instead, the program "diverts" them, or links them, with resources in the mental health system.

Diversion can only happen before you have a trial. Ask your lawyer, duty counsel, a Court Support Worker or a member of your support network to help refer you for diversion. The Crown has the authority to decide whether or not you are right for a diversion program.

To be diverted, the following conditions must be met:

- The offence you are charged with must be a minor one.
- You must volunteer to be diverted.
- The Crown must decide you are right for a diversion program.
- You must agree to follow a treatment plan that has been developed especially for you.

Psychiatrist

A psychiatrist is a medical doctor who has special training in assessing and treating mental illness. A psychiatrist can:

- prescribe medications to treat symptoms of mental illness
- see people for therapy or counselling
- assess people who may have a mental illness. One type of assessment is a forensic assessment. A **forensic assessment** is for the court. Please read the section "Getting a forensic assessment" on page 16 for more information.

Nurse

Nurses look after the daily needs of people who need medical help. They monitor patients, give emergency care, help people with hygiene and other activities of daily living, and much more. Nurses work in jails, hospitals and community agencies. Sometimes nurses visit a person's home. Nurses are usually part of the **interdisciplinary team**. This is the team of professionals involved in assessing and caring for you once you are in the forensic mental health system.

Psychologist

A psychologist has specialized knowledge of mental health problems. Psychologists often give tests to find out how people are functioning in areas such as intelligence and personality. They can test to assess brain function. Psychologists can also see people for therapy and counselling. A psychologist might be part of the team involved in assessing and caring for you.

Social worker

A social worker can help you find housing, get financial support and contact other community supports. Social workers also provide therapy and can organize and supervise visits with your family or others. Social workers are usually part of the team involved in assessing and caring for you. Ask your nurse or psychiatrist if there is a social worker on your team.

Recreation therapist

Recreation therapists help people to spend their free time in healthy ways. They help people to exercise their bodies by playing sports and keeping fit. They help people to exercise their minds by playing games and taking part in social activities. Recreation therapists are sometimes part of the team involved in assessing and caring for you. Ask your nurse or psychiatrist if there is a recreation therapist on your team.

Occupational therapist

Occupational therapists (OTS) can help you with everything from daily tasks to gaining employment skills. They help you to see your strengths and work on your weaknesses. OTS are sometimes part of the team involved in assessing and caring for you. Ask your nurse or psychiatrist if you have an occupational therapist on your team.

Patient advocates and rights advisers

Some Ontario hospitals have patient advocates. A patient advocate can help you make informed decisions about your care, treatment and legal rights. A patient advocate can also help you find lawyers and apply for Legal Aid.

Rights advisers give confidential advice about legal rights to people who are receiving psychiatric services.

The Psychiatric Patient Advocate Office (PPAO) offers these two services. The full range of services of the PPAO is not available in all Ontario hospitals. You can get in touch with a patient advocate or rights adviser in one of these ways:

- Call the PPAO at 1 800 578-2343.
- Visit the PPAO website at www.ppao.gov.on.ca to find out if there are services in your hospital.
- Visit a PPAO office in person. There are nine offices in Ontario. You can find the office nearest you on the website.
- If you do not have access to a telephone and you are not allowed to leave the hospital unit, ask one of the staff members to contact the PPAO office for you.

3 What happens inside the forensic mental health system?

The *Criminal Code of Canada* and the *Mental Health Act*

The rules for Canada's criminal justice system are set out in the *Criminal Code of Canada*. The mental health system in Ontario must also follow the *Mental Health Act*.

People working in the forensic mental health system must balance the rights and needs of an "accused" person (that is, the person charged with an offence) with the rights and needs of the public.

> At every stage, from assessment to absolute discharge, people working in the forensic mental health system must ensure your need for help and your rights are respected. You, and the people working with you, also have a responsibility to the public's need for safety.

How do people enter the forensic mental health system?

Police make the community safe and enforce the law. When someone calls the police because of something you did, the police must decide what to do:

- charge you with an offence and take you to jail
- take you to the hospital to be assessed
- release you without charges.

In choosing what to do, the police will talk to you and others involved to find out what happened. They will then:

- decide if they think you have committed a crime
- decide if they think you have a serious mental illness
- think about the safety of the community.

If the police think that you have a mental illness, they may take you to a hospital. You may still be charged with a crime.

Some people do not want to stay in the hospital. The *Mental Health Act* has strict rules about when people can be hospitalized against their will. If the rules are not met, you cannot be forced to stay in the hospital.

If you do not wish to stay in the hospital, and the rules of the *Mental Health Act* do not apply to you, the police must decide what to do next. If the police believe you have committed a crime, they may arrest you and take you to a jail or detention centre.

What happens after a person is arrested?

If you are arrested, you should contact a lawyer as soon as you can. To find a lawyer privately:

- look in the phone book under "Lawyers," or
- call the Law Society of Upper Canada's Lawyer Referral Service at 1 800 268-8326, or 416 947-3330 within the Greater Toronto Area, for a referral free of charge.

LEGAL AID

If you do not have the money to pay for a lawyer, you can apply for Legal Aid. Legal Aid is a program sponsored by the government of Ontario. It ensures that people who do not have money can still have a lawyer. Based on your financial situation, you may not have to pay anything, or you may have to pay only a small part of the cost of Legal Aid.

You have to apply for Legal Aid. If you are not in jail or in the hospital, you have to apply in person at a Legal Aid clinic. If you are in the hospital, contact the patient advocate or rights adviser to get help applying for Legal Aid. Applying involves filling out an application form and giving some financial information. If you are approved for Legal Aid, you will get what is called a Legal Aid certificate. You can then contact a lawyer of your choice as long as that lawyer will accept Legal Aid certificates.

For information about applying for Legal Aid:

- call 416 598-0200 in Toronto, or
- call 1 800 668-8258 outside the Greater Toronto Area, or
- visit the Legal Aid website at www.legalaid.on.ca.

Read the section "Patient advocates and rights advisers" on page 10 for information about contacting a patient advocate.

Being held in the hospital

If you go to the hospital (either with police, with family or friends, or by yourself), a doctor will assess you. If the doctor thinks that you need a longer inpatient psychiatric assessment, the doctor will fill out a Form 1. This form is called "Application by Physician for Psychiatric Assessment."

A doctor can only fill out a **Form 1** under conditions set out in the Ontario *Mental Health Act*. Find out more about these conditions from a lawyer, a patient advocate or a rights adviser.

If a doctor fills out a Form 1, you can be kept in the hospital for up to 72 hours, even if it is against your will. This is called involuntary admission. You must have another psychiatric assessment within 72 hours after a Form 1 is filled out. The doctor must decide if you still meet the conditions for **involuntary admission**.

If the doctor believes that you do not meet the conditions, you can no longer be held in the hospital without your consent. If the police have charged you with a crime, you may be brought to jail or to court.

If the doctor believes that you still meet the criteria for involuntary admission, the doctor will fill out a **Form 3**. This form is called "Certificate of Involuntary Admission." A person can be held in the hospital on a Form 3 for up to two weeks. If the doctor believes that you still meet the criteria for involuntary admission, a **Form 4**: "Certificate of Renewal" will be used. A Form 4 can be used for as long as you continue to meet the criteria for involuntary admission.

Getting a forensic assessment

If your lawyer, Crown counsel or the judge believes that mental illness was a factor in the crime you are accused of, that person will ask for a **forensic assessment**. This assessment is designed to answer specific questions, which are set out in the *Criminal Code of Canada*.

You cannot be sent for a forensic assessment just because you seem to be ill. Evidence must be given to the court to support an order for a forensic assessment.

Most often, the forensic assessment is ordered to find out:

• whether you are Fit to Stand Trial, or
• whether you are criminally responsible for your actions.

Other special types of forensic assessment include pre-sentence assessments and dangerous or long-term offender assessments.

Determining Fitness to Stand Trial

Your lawyer, Crown counsel or the judge will ask for a forensic assessment if they think that mental illness might prevent you from taking part in the court proceedings. The court proceedings include hearings, trials and any other part of the legal process. People who are able to take part in the proceedings are referred to as "Fit." People who are not able to take part are referred to as "Unfit." The issue of fitness can be raised at any time from arrest to sentencing.

The Criminal Code of Canada **states that you are Unfit if, because of a mental illness:**

you cannot understand the nature, object or consequences of what happens in court,

OR

you are unable to communicate with and instruct your lawyer.

Having a mental illness does not necessarily mean that you are Unfit to Stand Trial. The court decides whether you are Fit or Unfit. Psychiatrists and other mental health professionals do forensic assessments to help the court make this decision.

To decide that you are **Fit to Stand Trial**, the judge must believe that you are able to do the following:

- You must be able to describe the roles of the people in a courtroom, such as the Crown counsel, the defence counsel (your lawyer) and the judge.
- You must have a general understanding of what happens in court. For instance, you must understand what the possible verdicts (or outcomes) are and what an oath is.
- You must be able to instruct your lawyer and take part in your own defence.

Fitness to Stand Trial and Treatment Orders

If you are Unfit to Stand Trial, a judge might order you to be treated with medication to make you Fit. This is called a Treatment Order. If you are under a **Treatment Order** you must take the prescribed medication. If you refuse to take medication, it may be given to you in an injection or by mouth.

If you are under a Treatment Order, you will stay in the hospital, or under some circumstances the court may agree to you receiving care in the community. The order usually lasts up to 60 days. If you are Fit by the time the order expires, you will go back to court to face your charges. If you are still Unfit when the order expires, you will likely be placed under the authority of the Ontario Review Board (ORB).

Determining Criminal Responsibility

Your lawyer, Crown counsel or the judge will ask for a forensic assessment if any one of them thinks that mental illness might have affected your actions at the time you committed a crime. If you did not understand what you were doing or did not know it was wrong because of mental illness, you could be found **"Not Criminally Responsible"** (NCR).

Having a mental illness does not necessarily mean that you are NCR. The court decides whether you are NCR. Psychiatrists and other mental health professionals do forensic assessments to help the court make this decision.

> *The Criminal Code of Canada* states that you are "Not Criminally Responsible" (NCR) for an offence if a mental disorder prevents you from:
>
> appreciating the nature of your actions
>
> OR
>
> knowing that your actions were wrong.

If you are found NCR, it means that the court believes you did do something illegal. However, because of your mental illness, the court finds that you should not be held responsible under the law. NCR used to be called "Not Guilty by Reason of Insanity." You may have heard people talking about the "insanity defence" or "pleading insanity" on television and in the movies. In Canada, we now call this "Not Criminally Responsible."

NCR refers to your mental state only at the time an offence occurred.

What happens during a forensic assessment?

You might be assessed by a forensic psychiatrist in jail, at the court-house or in a hospital. Usually, a forensic psychiatrist will talk to you and ask questions. The forensic psychiatrist may also interview members of your family and support network. There may also be medical and psychological testing. Some assessments (usually for

Fitness) occur right in the courthouse. Some cities have a Mental Health Court that deals only with cases where mental illness is a factor.

Some courthouses have a Court Support Program. If your offence is considered minor you may be eligible for "diversion" out of the criminal justice system. The program will help you find support and treatment in the community.

Assessments in the forensic unit of a psychiatric hospital are called inpatient assessments. If you are in a jail or detention centre and the court orders an inpatient assessment for you, you will be transferred directly from the detention centre. You will still be "in custody," that is, under the control of the court, during the assessment. You will be returned to the detention centre or go directly to court when the assessment is done.

During the assessment, you might see psychiatrists, nurses, social workers, recreation therapists and psychologists. They are your assessors.

After the assessment is done, the forensic psychiatrist will usually write a report for the court. The psychiatrist or any other assessor might also testify in court.

A psychiatrist who is doing a forensic assessment is working for the court to help answer questions about your mental condition. The psychiatrist is not for or against you. Forensic psychiatrists simply try to find out all they can, so that they can give an informed opinion to the court. The forensic psychiatrist who assesses you will not provide you with treatment, but may take steps to see that you are offered treatment. Whatever you tell a forensic psychiatrist and the other professionals assessing you is not confidential. The assessors can report any information that you give them to the court.

Refusing to take part in a forensic assessment

You have the right to refuse to take part in some or all of the assessment. Sometimes your friends or family members will be asked for information about you. They have the right to refuse to answer questions too. Any information they do give could also be used in court. In some cases, family members decide to contact the assessors on their own. They do this if they feel they have information that will help the assessors understand your situation better.

Even if you decide not to take part in the assessment, the forensic psychiatrist must still report to the court. He or she must respond to the question the court has asked. For example, "Is this person Fit to Stand Trial?" or "Is this person criminally responsible?"

The forensic psychiatrist will report to the court using any available information, such as:

• police and hospital records
• information given by your friends, family or co-workers
• observations of you in the hospital.

The court's decision

Based on the forensic assessment, the judge will make a decision. If the court finds that you are Fit to Stand Trial, you will continue to face your charges in court.

If the court decides that you are Unfit or "Not Criminally Responsible" (NCR), the court may hold a disposition hearing to determine what will happen to you next. If the court does not hold a disposition hearing, you will be placed under the authority of the **Ontario Review Board** (ORB), who will then be responsible for holding the disposition hearing.

If you have been found NCR by the court, you will be given one of the following three orders at your disposition hearing:

• an absolute discharge
• a conditional discharge
• a detention order.

(All of these terms are described in Chapter 4.)

If you have been found Unfit by the court, you may be given a conditional discharge or a detention order at your disposition hearing, but you will not be able to get an absolute discharge.

If you are given a conditional discharge or a detention order at your disposition hearing, the ORB will make longer-term decisions about what level of security and types of "privileges" you will be given (these are explained on pages 29–30). You will continue to have disposition hearings with the ORB once a year as long as you are under the authority of the ORB. We will talk more about this in the next chapter.

4 The Ontario Review Board (ORB)

What is the Ontario Review Board (ORB)?

If you are placed under the authority of the Ontario Review Board (ORB) after you have been found Unfit to Stand Trial (Unfit) or Not Criminally Responsible (NCR), you must follow the orders of the ORB the same way you must follow the orders of a judge.

The ORB is a panel, usually made up of:

- a psychiatrist
- a mental health professional, such as a psychiatrist or psychologist
- a lawyer
- a person from the community with a background in mental health
- a chairperson who is either a senior lawyer or a retired judge.

This panel is responsible for making ongoing decisions about you. The members review your situation regularly. They decide things such as:

- what level of security you should have
- whether you will go to a hospital
- which hospital you will go to
- when you can have privileges to go back into the community
- what kind of supervision and support you should have in the community.

You will be referred to as "the accused."

When will I have my first hearing?

If the court had a disposition hearing, and you did not obtain an absolute discharge during that hearing, you will have your first ORB **hearing** within 90 days. If the court did not have a disposition hearing, you will have your first hearing with the ORB sooner— within 45 days.

After your first ORB hearing, you will have one ORB hearing every year. On rare occasions, it is possible that you could have a special early hearing if there has been a major change in your situation or your health.

What happens in the ORB hearing?

Hearings usually take place in a boardroom or special hearing room in the hospital. In more rural areas, a person may have to travel to get to the ORB hearing. ORB hearings are less formal than courtroom proceedings, but they still have rules that must be followed.

You will sit in front of the ORB panel with your lawyer. A Crown counsel, your psychiatrist and a representative from the hospital will also be there. Most of the time, ORB hearings are open to the public, so your family and friends can attend.

The panel hears evidence from you and your lawyer, your psychiatrist and sometimes other people, such as a family member or another specialist. The hospital submits a report to the ORB giving your history and progress. You and your lawyer get a copy of this report.

The court found me Not Criminally Responsible (NCR). What can the ORB decide about me?

If you have been found NCR, your ORB hearing can have one of three outcomes:

1. The *Criminal Code of Canada* says that the ORB must grant you an **absolute discharge** if you are not "a significant threat to the safety of the public." Absolute discharge means that you are no longer under the authority of the ORB. You are free to live where and how you wish within the limits of the law. An important legal case in 1999 clarified the meaning of "significant threat." It means "a real risk of physical or psychological harm to members of the public that is serious in the sense of going beyond the merely trivial or annoying" [Winko v. British Columbia (Forensic Psychiatric Institute)].

2. You may be given a **conditional discharge.** This means that you are no longer required to live in the hospital. However, you must follow the conditions set by the ORB. These might include reporting to the hospital and giving urine samples to test for alcohol or other drug use. You must continue to attend annual ORB hearings. If you do not follow the conditions set for you, the police could return you to the hospital. The ORB believes that you would be a significant threat to the public if you were not following the conditions.

3. You are subject to a **detention order.** This means that the ORB believes you would be a "significant threat" to the public if you were released. You remain under the authority of the ORB and you will have another ORB hearing in one year.

The court found me Unfit to Stand Trial. What can the ORB decide about me?

If you have been found Unfit to Stand Trial, your ORB hearing can have one of three outcomes:

1. You are found **Fit to Stand Trial.** The ORB may decide that you are now Fit and able to face your charges in court. In this case, you will no longer be under the authority of the ORB. You will be sent back to court.

2. You remain **Unfit** to Stand Trial and get a conditional discharge. This means that you are no longer required to live in the hospital. However, you must follow the conditions set by the ORB. These might include reporting to the hospital and giving urine samples to test for alcohol or other drug use. If you do not follow the conditions set for you, the police could return you to the hospital. If your doctor decides, at any time during the year, that you are now Fit, she or he can contact the ORB for a hearing. If the Board finds you Fit, you will return to court.

3. You remain Unfit to Stand Trial and you are subject to a detention order. This means that you are still under the authority of the ORB and may have to stay in the hospital. You will have another ORB hearing in one year unless your doctor believes you have become Fit before that time.

What happens after the hearing?

After your ORB hearing, the ORB will make a disposition. This is a decision, or order. The disposition states:

• whether you should be placed in the community, with regular hospital visits
• whether you will be hospitalized
• what level of security you require
• what types of privileges you can have
• what conditions you must follow over the next year.

Some examples of **conditions** placed on you might include:

• giving random urine samples to see if you have been using alcohol or other drugs
• making regular visits to your case worker or psychiatrist
• not carrying or owning weapons.

Also, you must follow the rules and regulations of the hospital unit you are connected to.

How long can the ORB keep me in the hospital?

If you have been found Unfit to Stand Trial, or Not Criminally Responsible (NCR), there is no set date for release the way there is with a jail sentence. *You may have to spend longer in the hospital than you would have spent in jail if you had been found guilty in court,* or the time may be shorter.

What hospital will I go to?

You will usually go to a hospital with a forensic program. The ORB will choose the hospital, based on where you lived before you were arrested and what level of security you require. The ORB may also try to place you close to family, cultural supports or treatments that could help you.

ONTARIO HOSPITALS WITH FORENSIC PROGRAMS

- Centre for Addiction and Mental Health (Toronto)
- Lakehead Psychiatric Hospital (Thunder Bay)
- Mental Health Centre, Penetanguishene (Ontario's only maximum security unit)
- North Bay Regional Health Centre (formerly North Bay Psychiatric Hospital)
- Providence Care Mental Health Services (formerly Kingston Psychiatric Hospital)
- Royal Ottawa Hospital (including the former Brockville Psychiatric Hospital)

- St. Joseph's Healthcare Hamilton
- St. Joseph's Regional Mental Health Care London (formerly London Psychiatric Hospital and St. Thomas Psychiatric Hospital)
- Syl Apps Youth Centre—Kinark Child and Family Services (This facility is for teenagers under the age of 16. Older teens go through the same process as adults do.)
- Ontario Shores Centre for Mental Health Sciences (formerly Whitby Mental Health Centre).

There are three levels of security in hospital units in the forensic mental health system: maximum, secure or general security. Some people must work their way from the most secure (maximum) to the least secure (general). Others will be placed on a general unit right away. The level of security you require is related to the risk you present to the community, and also to your health needs.

Privileges in my disposition

The ORB disposition will list the **privileges** you may have for up to one year, or until your next ORB hearing. Privileges involve increasing amounts of freedom and responsibility, such as walking on the hospital grounds or visiting or living in the community. The doctor and interdisciplinary team will decide what level of privilege you will start with and work toward, as long as the privileges are allowed by your ORB disposition.

The team may take away, or suspend, privileges if you do not use them properly or do not follow unit rules. The team will also suspend privileges if they are concerned that you are a danger to yourself or others.

If your disposition allows you a privilege in the company of an **approved person**, a family member or friend can apply. That person must have a criminal background check and an interview with your team. An approved person must follow the rules of your disposition. Talk to your team about who would make a good approved person.

If you use your privileges without problems and follow the unit rules, the team will usually recommend at your yearly ORB hearing that your privileges be increased.

Preparing for an ORB hearing

Over the year, you will work with your psychiatrist and interdisciplinary team to improve or maintain your mental health. Your goal is to show that you can use your highest level of privileges without problems. Before your annual ORB hearing, the team will meet to discuss your progress.

Each year, the hospital will write a report for the ORB, outlining:

- the things that have gone well and anything that has not gone so well over the past year
- the privileges and conditions recommended by the team for the next year
- your expectations and hopes for the next year, if you have told the team what they are.

Many forensic programs use **risk assessments** to help them decide on privileges and recommendations to the ORB. "Risk" refers to the likelihood that you will commit another offence. Usually, the forensic mental health system is interested in your risk for committing a violent act. Most risk assessments involve an interview with a psychologist or psychiatrist, or with other mental health professionals.

You can choose not to take part in the interview. The assessor might also read your hospital files and talk to members of your family and support network.

How does the ORB make its decisions?

Decisions are made by a majority vote. The Board considers four things:

1. Are you a risk to members of the public?

2. How is your mental health now? How has it been over the past year?

3. How well integrated into society are you? For instance, do you have good connections to any friends or family? Could you do a job or be a volunteer? Do you have any income? Could you successfully live outside of the hospital?

4. Do you have any other needs that should be considered?

Given the answers to each of these questions, the ORB has to decide what will be the "least onerous and least restrictive" disposition. This means that the ORB has to give you the most freedom possible. At the same time, the ORB must keep in mind your safety, your treatment needs and the safety of the public.

Appealing an ORB decision

If you believe that the ORB has made an unfair decision, there is a process of appeal. This involves the Court of Appeal, which is part of the criminal justice system. You cannot appeal an ORB decision just because you don't like it. You have to be able to argue that the decision was not made fairly or lawfully. Talk to your lawyer to find out more about whether you have grounds to appeal.

5 Accepting or refusing treatment in the forensic mental health system

Even if you have been hospitalized against your will, you cannot be forced to accept treatment unless:

- the doctor signs a certificate saying that you are incapable of consenting or refusing, or
- you have been found Unfit to Stand Trial, and the judge has ordered treatment to enable you to become Fit to Stand Trial or help you stay Fit to Stand Trial.

Incapacity to accept or refuse treatment

When a doctor feels that you are too ill to understand your condition, or the consequences of accepting or refusing treatment, the doctor can complete a form that makes a finding of incapacity. This is what happens:

- A doctor completes a form, making a finding of incapacity.
- The hospital tells the rights adviser.
- The rights adviser visits you and advises you of your legal right to challenge the doctor's finding.

- If you *do not challenge* the doctor's finding of incapacity, a **substitute decision maker** (SDM) is named.
- If you decide to *challenge* the doctor's finding, a hearing with the **Consent and Capacity Board** will be started within seven days.

Substitute decision makers (SDMs)

Usually, a substitute decision maker (SDM) is someone who is related to you. If no one in your family is willing or able to take on this role, someone from the Public Guardian's office will be named as your SDM. The SDM makes treatment decisions for you. If the SDM consents to the treatment advised by your doctor, you will receive that treatment, even if it is against your will.

It is the psychiatrist's responsibility to keep assessing your capacity to consent to treatment. When you do understand that you have a mental illness and you know what will happen if you accept or refuse treatment, the SDM can step down. Then you can make your own decisions about treatment.

Going to the Consent and Capacity Board

If you challenge your doctor's finding of incapacity to consent to treatment, you will have a hearing with the Consent and Capacity Board. The Board is made up of one, three or five impartial psychiatrists, lawyers and members of the public. They follow the rules in the *Mental Health Act,* the *Health Care Consent Act,* the *Substitute Decisions Act* and the *Long Term Care Act.*

Your psychiatrist must give the Board evidence that you are incapable of consenting to or refusing treatment. Everyone involved in the hearing can have a lawyer present, call witnesses or bring documents.

If the Consent and Capacity Board finds that you are incapable of consenting to or refusing treatment, a substitute decision maker (SDM) will be named.

If the Board finds that you are capable of consenting to or refusing treatment, you now have the right to accept or refuse treatment. Before you do, talk to the team members that are taking care of you about your concerns. Discuss treatment options with them.

6 Living in a forensic mental health setting

Living under the authority of the Ontario Review Board (ORB) can be hard. You are trying to cope with a mental illness. You are dealing with the stress of the event that brought you into the system. Your freedom may be restricted. You may feel frightened, or powerless, or lonely. And of course in a hospital, you will find other people trying to cope with problems of their own, but many may have similar problems to yours.

Talking about your concerns is the best way to resolve them. You can talk to the members of your interdisciplinary team, such as your psychiatrist, nurse or social worker. They will help you understand why restrictions have been imposed on you. You can also make a plan with your team to increase your privileges over time.

The controls on your behaviour and freedom are meant to ensure safety for you, other patients and the community while you are improving your health.

Where can I turn for help if I feel I am being treated unfairly?

If you cannot resolve a problem with your team, there are several people you can turn to. You, a family member or someone from your personal support network can contact one of the following people:

- Most hospitals have client/patient relations co-ordinators. Ask any member of your team how to contact them. You can ask questions, make suggestions, or voice concerns about your care at the hospital.
- Ask any member of your team how to contact the director of the forensic program at your hospital.
- Contact the Psychiatric Patient Advocate Office (PPAO) at 1 800 578-2343 or go to the website at www.ppao.gov.on.ca. Patient advocates do not work for the hospital.
- Some hospitals have a Family Resource Centre or Family Council.

Getting help for other problems

Many people in the forensic mental health system face problems in their lives other than mental illness. Forensic and general psychiatric hospitals often have programs to help with:

- drug and alcohol abuse
- family problems
- language difficulties
- social skills
- sexual problems
- financial problems
- physical health problems.

Based on your level of security, you may also be able to attend community programs outside of the hospital. Talk to your team about options and ideas for you.

Language and interpreters

If you are not comfortable speaking or reading English, or if you are deaf, ask for an interpreter. There is no cost to you. Courts and hospitals in big cities can usually book an interpreter for interviews and meetings. In rural areas, it might take longer to get an interpreter.

Human rights in the forensic mental health system

Some personal freedoms may be restricted while you are in the forensic mental health system. However, the Constitution ensures that all Canadians are protected against discrimination. Under the *Charter of Rights and Freedoms*, you have the right to be free from discrimination based on:

- race
- gender
- sexual orientation
- mental or physical ability
- age
- religion.

You have many other rights protected by the *Charter of Rights and Freedoms*, whatever your forensic status. Speak to your lawyer about those rights.

Your rights as a patient under the authority of the Ontario Review Board (ORB)

1. Although rules and restrictions may be imposed on you while you are in the forensic mental health system, you have the right to be treated with respect. In turn, you will be expected to treat staff and co-patients with respect.

2. You have the right to decide about your treatment unless you are:

   - deemed incapable of consenting to or refusing treatment, or
   - subject to a Treatment Order.

3. You have the right to be involved in and asked about your treatment and care even if you are not capable of consenting to or refusing treatment.

4. You have the right to limited confidentiality. That means that, usually, only the people assessing and treating you will have access to information about you. However, there are many exceptions. Other people will have access to your information if:

   - you give your consent for others to have access to your information
   - the hospital has to share information with authorities such as the ORB, the courts or the police
   - the staff treating you have a duty to warn or protect other people.

5. You have the right to refuse to take part in a forensic assessment. However, keep in mind that the assessment will still take place using other available information.

6. You have the right to reasonable access to an interpreter.

7. You have the right to an ORB hearing once every year.

8. You have the right to be present at your ORB hearing unless you are a danger to yourself or others at the time of the hearing.

9. You have the right to speak or present evidence at your ORB hearing.

10. You have the right to a lawyer. You have the right to confidential communication with your lawyer.

11. You have a limited right to look at your clinical record. Talk to your psychiatrist or another member of your team about the limits to this right.

12. You have the right to contact with a spiritual adviser of your choice.

13. You have the right to a safe environment when you are staying on a forensic mental health unit in Ontario.

14. You have the right to vote if you are an eligible Canadian citizen.

15. You have the right to talk to a patient advocate, client relations co-ordinator or family advocate. You have the right to be informed of your rights.

7 Family, friends and the forensic mental health system

If someone in your family or your circle of friends has a mental illness, you may have already gone through a lot of distress. It is even harder when that person comes into conflict with the law. You may have made the painful decision to call the police yourself, when you saw someone you love doing something wrong or frightening.

Why does it seem so hard to get help?

People who have a mental illness often do not know that they are ill. You may have already tried to get your loved one to go into a hospital or to see a doctor, without success.

Sometimes people call the police, hoping that this is a way to get help. If the police believe that there has been a crime, they must act. That does not always mean that your loved one will go to the hospital and get treated.

In Canada, the people who report a possible crime do not press charges themselves, even if they are the victims. It is the police who press charges. Once you call the police, you cannot say that you want to "press charges" or "drop charges."

The rules in the *Criminal Code of Canada* and the *Mental Health Act* may seem frustrating at times. However, they are meant to protect the rights and freedoms of all people, including people who have a mental illness. Sometimes family and friends do not want the same thing as the person with the mental illness. The mental health system can only force people to be hospitalized in situations when someone is very unwell, usually when people are a threat to themselves or to public safety.

Supporting someone in the forensic mental health system

When a friend or loved one has to go to jail or the hospital, you can be left with mixed emotions—fear, guilt, anger, frustration, relief. All of these feelings are normal.

You have to decide how much support you are willing or able to give. Talk to the psychiatrist or social worker about the different ways you can support your loved one.

Look after yourself. Some people find it helps to talk to a family doctor, a psychologist or psychiatrist, a spiritual counsellor or a trusted friend.

Some hospitals have services that help the family and friends of patients to get information and support. Also, look in local newspapers, on bulletin boards and on the Internet for groups in your community.

Visiting a jail or hospital

Visiting someone in jail or on the forensic unit of a hospital is easier if you know what to expect.

Call the jail or hospital unit ahead of time. Find out:

• the visiting hours
• the rules about bringing gifts such as food, cigarettes, money or clothing
• the rules for bringing children
• anything else you need to know before you visit.

A forensic unit in a hospital must make sure the environment is safe for everyone. To ensure this, your bags or clothing will be searched. You will have to show photo identification before being allowed to visit.

Seeing someone in a forensic unit of a hospital can be upsetting. Your loved one may be experiencing symptoms of mental illness. Or the person may be sedated (sleepy or sluggish because of medication). Knowing what to expect will make your visit easier.

8 Leaving the forensic mental health system

Ending the relationship with the Ontario Review Board (ORB)

You are no longer under the authority of the Ontario Review Board (ORB) when:

- you have been granted an absolute discharge, or
- you have been found Fit to Stand Trial and returned to court.

At this point, you no longer have to stay in contact with mental health professionals. However, most people find it is better to stay connected to a hospital or community mental health services.

Staying connected to community resources

Many people who are no longer under the authority of the ORB still need some help. This support can help you avoid coming back into the forensic mental health system.

If you are taking medication to help treat the symptoms of mental illness, you must keep seeing your doctor. Staying connected to a mental health resource can also help you deal with challenges you might face while living in the community.

Conclusion

The forensic mental health system can be confusing for patients and those who love them. We hope this guide helps you to understand the system better. Every person's situation is unique—sometimes, rules and procedures are used that are different from the ones we have written about here. Also, some services offered at hospitals in big cities are not always available in smaller communities. If you have questions that this guide does not answer, talk to your lawyer, doctor or another professional in the forensic mental health system. Resources for further information have also been listed at the back of this guide.

Glossary

absolute discharge: A person is no longer subject to the authority of the Ontario Review Board (ORB). The person is free to live where he or she likes within the limits of the law.

approved person: A person who has applied for and been accepted as the person who will escort you on privileges and who agrees to follow the rules and restrictions in your disposition.

conditional discharge: Also known as "discharge subject to conditions." A person is still under the authority of the Ontario Review Board (ORB), but is allowed to live in the community. The person must, however, follow the conditions laid out in the disposition. Examples of conditions that are often enforced are abstaining from alcohol or other drugs, submitting to random drug screens and having regular meetings with a psychiatrist or other mental health professional.

conditions: Rules that must be followed in a disposition order.

Consent and Capacity Board: An independent panel established by the Ontario government that conducts different types of hearings, including deciding on a person's capacity to consent to or refuse treatment.

Court Support Program: A program that exists in some courts to help people become connected with psychiatric services and community resources.

criminal justice system: The system that deals with people accused of and convicted of crimes.

criminal responsibility: A court may decide that a person did commit a crime, but find that person Not Criminally Responsible (NCR). A court finds a person NCR when, because of a mental illness, that person could not appreciate the nature of his or her actions or did not know that the actions were wrong. However, simply having a mental disorder does not make a person NCR.

detention order: A person on a detention order is still under the authority of the Ontario Review Board (ORB). Some people on detention orders have the privilege of living in the community. The psychiatrist and interdisciplinary team have the right to allow or deny any privilege listed on the disposition.

disposition: A decision the Ontario Review Board (ORB) makes after having a hearing. A disposition details where a person must go, for example, which hospital, facility or doctor the person must remain connected to. A disposition also details what level of security the person will be subject to (maximum, secure or general) and the privileges and conditions that apply for the next year.

disposition hearing: This is where a person who has been found Unfit to Stand Trial (Unfit) or Not Criminally Responsible (NCR) may be given:

- an absolute discharge (only available for those who are NCR)
- a conditional discharge
- a detention order.

The first disposition hearing could happen in the court or with the Ontario Review Board (ORB), if the court decides not to conduct this hearing. All subsequent disposition hearings, if there are any, will be conducted by the ORB.

If the court chooses to hold a disposition hearing, the ORB will then be required to hold another disposition hearing within 90 days. The only exception is when a person found NCR is given an absolute discharge. In that case, there are no further decisions to be made because the person is no longer involved with the forensic mental health system.

If the court chooses not to hold a disposition hearing, the ORB must hold a disposition hearing within 45 days of the finding of NCR or Unfit.

After the first disposition hearing, you will typically have one ORB disposition hearing a year for as long as you remain under the authority of the ORB.

diversion: Minor charges are dropped, or stayed, if the accused person agrees to follow an individually tailored treatment plan. The Crown decides whether an accused person will be diverted. The defence counsel, duty counsel and court support worker can help a person look into the possibility of diversion.

dual diagnosis: A person who has both a mental illness and an intellectual disability (also known as a "developmental delay" or "mental retardation").

Fit to Stand Trial: The ability of a person to understand what happens in court and what might result from the proceedings, and also the person's ability to communicate with his or her lawyer. A person is declared Unfit to Stand Trial ("Unfit") if a mental illness stops that person from understanding the nature, object or consequences of the events that happen in court, or if that illness stops the person from being able to communicate with and instruct his or her lawyer. Simply having a mental disorder does not make a person Unfit.

forensic: Connected to the law or the courts.

forensic assessment: The systematic evaluation of an issue, such as Fitness to Stand Trial or Criminal Responsibility. The results of the assessment are made into a report for the court.

forensic mental health system: The system that deals with people who have a mental illness (including those with a dual diagnosis) and who have come into contact with the law.

Form 1: "Application by Physician for Psychiatric Assessment." A legal document that comes from the *Mental Health Act*. If a doctor thinks that you have a mental disorder and you are going to harm yourself or someone else, or that you can't look after yourself, the doctor may fill out a Form 1. (Talk to a psychiatrist, lawyer or patient advocate for more information about the criteria for a Form 1.) Once this form is signed, you can be kept in hospital for up to 72 hours, even if it is against your will.

Form 3: "Certificate of Involuntary Admission." Once you are in hospital on a Form 1, a physician must assess you again within 72 hours. If a doctor thinks you still meet the criteria for involuntary admission to hospital, the doctor may fill out a Form 3. After a Form 3 has been signed, you can be kept in hospital for up to two weeks.

Form 4: "Certificate of Renewal." If a doctor thinks you still meet the criteria for involuntary admission to hospital after a Form 3 expires, the doctor may fill out a Form 4. The doctor can use a Form 4 for as long as you meet the criteria for involuntary admission to hospital.

hearing: A forum where legal proceedings are held. Hearings decide such things as whether a psychiatric assessment is needed, whether a person should be granted bail or what a guilty person's sentence should be.

interdisciplinary team: A group of people who are involved in your forensic assessment, or in your care once you are in the forensic mental health system. This group might include people from some or all of the following professions: nursing, medicine, social work, psychology, recreation therapy or occupational therapy.

involuntary admission: When you are kept in hospital even if it is against your will.

mental health system: The system that assesses and cares for people with mental health problems.

Not Criminally Responsible (NCR): See Criminal responsibility.

Ontario Review Board (ORB): People who are found Unfit, or Not Criminally Responsible (NCR), are placed under the authority of the ORB. They will have a hearing within 45 days or 90 days of the initial finding and then once a year after that. The ORB panel decides what kind of privileges a person will have for the year, where that person will go and what level of security is needed.

privileges: The amount and kind of freedoms a person may have during the year when that person is under the authority of the Ontario Review Board (ORB). Having a stable mental status, following the rules and using privileges without problems usually leads to more privileges. The psychiatrist has the right to allow, refuse or revoke (cancel) any privilege listed on the ORB's disposition, based on that psychiatrist's assessment of the safety of the person and the public. The goal of privileges is to help people become re-integrated into society.

risk assessment: Ways of assessing the likelihood of future problem behaviour, usually violence.

substitute decision maker (sdm): Person who is appointed to decide on treatment for a patient who has been found incapable of consenting to or refusing treatment. If no relative is willing or able to be the sdm, an independent organization called the Public Guardian and Trustee will be made the sdm.

Treatment Order: A time-limited order made by the court that permits people to be treated, even against their will. The purpose of a treatment order is to help make a person Fit to Stand Trial.

trial: A formal proceeding to decide a case by a court of law. A verdict of guilty, not guilty or Not Criminally Responsible (ncr) will be determined at a trial.

Unfit: See Fit to Stand Trial.

Where to go for more information

GENERAL INFORMATION

The **Canadian Mental Health Association**, Ontario, offers general information on mental health issues. Visit their website at www.ontario.cmha.ca or call 1 800 875-6213 or 416 977-5580 (in Toronto).

CENTRE FOR ADDICTION AND MENTAL HEALTH (CAMH)

The **Law and Mental Health Program website** provides information on the services offered, as well as a brief description of some important issues in forensic mental health:

Visit the CAMH website at www.camh.net and type "Law and Mental Health" in the search bar.

The **Family Council** supports the families of people who are involved with CAMH. The Family Council seeks to empower families by providing advocacy, support and information. Call 416 535-8501 ext. 6499 or 6490.

The **Family Resource Centre** is a program of the Family Council, providing information and ongoing support to family members of those receiving mental health services at CAMH. Call 416 535-8501 ext. 4015.

CONSENT AND CAPACITY

For more information on the **Consent and Capacity Board**, visit
their website at www.ccboard.on.ca.

DUAL DIAGNOSIS

Note: Although dual diagnosis sometimes also means a combination
of mental illness and drug or alcohol addiction, these services are
only for people who have a dual diagnosis of mental illness and
intellectual disability.

Dual Diagnosis Program, Centre for Addiction and Mental Health
(CAMH), 416 535-8501 ext. 7809. This service is for people who have
both a mental illness and an intellectual disability (also known as
"developmental delay" or "mental retardation"). The service includes
phone consultation, time-limited assessment, treatment and supports
for consumers, their support networks and their service providers.

Concerned Parents of Toronto Inc. provides support and information
to families to help them support those with a dual diagnosis.
Phone them at 416 492-1468 or e-mail them at thejohnstons1@
sympatico.ca.

OTHER ORGANIZATIONS AND SERVICES

Family Association for Mental Health Everywhere (FAME): If
someone you care about has been diagnosed with a mental illness,
you can contact FAME at 416 207-5032 for more information.

Legal Aid Ontario will provide affordable legal counsel to those who are unable to pay regular legal fees. You can reach Legal Aid at 1 800 668-8258 or 416 598-0200 (in Toronto), or visit their website at www.legalaid.on.ca.

Mood Disorders Association of Ontario has expertise in mood disorders such as bipolar disorder or major depressive disorder. If someone you care about has been diagnosed with a mood disorder, contact the Mood Disorders Association of Ontario at 1 888 486-8236 or 416 486-8046 (in Toronto) for information.

Psychiatric Patient Advocate Office (PPAO): The PPAO has created a few different booklets on issues to do with psychiatric clients and the law. Call PPAO at 1 800 578-2343 or 416 327-7000 (in Toronto), or visit their website at www.ppao.gov.on.ca.

Schizophrenia Society of Ontario provides family-based advocacy and can be reached at 1 800 449-6367 or 416 449-6830 (in Toronto), or visit their website at www.schizophrenia.on.ca.

OTHER GUIDES IN THIS SERIES

Addiction

Anxiety Disorders

Bipolar Disorder

Cognitive-Behavioural Therapy

Concurrent Substance Use and Mental Health Disorders

Couple Therapy

Depressive Illness

First Episode Psychosis

Obsessive-Compulsive Disorder

Women, Abuse and Trauma Therapy

Women and Psychosis

To order these and other camh publications,
contact Sales and Distribution:

Tel: 1 800 661-1111
Toronto: 416 595-6059
E-mail: publications@camh.net
Online store: http://store.camh.net